HEARING LOSS AND WINNING SOLUTIONS

STRATEGIES
FOR
The Hearing-Impaired and Their Families and Friends

By
Professor Nancy Shuster, M.A.T., M.Ed.

Hearing Loss and Winning Solutions
Copyright ©2004 by Professor Nancy Shuster

SLR Publishing Inc.
8310 Excalibur Circle Q7
Naples, Florida 34108
E-mail Nshu4@aol.com

All rights reserved. This book or parts of this book may not be reproduced in any form without written permission from the publisher.

WARNING AND DISCLAIMER: Every effort has been made to make this book as accurate as possible. It is published with the understanding that the publisher and the author shall have neither liability nor responsibility to any person with respect to any loss or damages arising from the information contained in this book.

ISBN: 0-9726730-0-8
Library of Congress Catalog Card Number: Pending

First Edition: April 2004

CONTENTS

Preface v
Acknowledgments vi
Notice to the Reader vii

Chapter 1 1
Defining the Problem
Solutions 4

Chapter 2 5
Emotional Reactions
Solutions 11

Chapter 3 13
Hearing Loss in Children
Solutions 16

Chapter 4 17
Hearing Aids
Solutions 22-23

Chapter 5 25
Assistive Listening Devices
Solutions 34

Chapter 6 35
Strategies that Work
Solutions 41-42

Chapter 7 43
Computers, E-mail, Internet
Solutions 46

iii

Chapter 8 47
Support Groups
Solutions 51

Chapter 9 53
Cochlear Implants
Solutions 58-59

Chapter 10 61
Future Research
Solutions 64

Appendix A 67
Product Comparisons

Appendix B 71
Americans with Disabilities Act

Appendix C 75
Captioned Telephones

Bibliography 80-81

Index 83-84

Ordering Forms 85-87

iv

PREFACE

Hearing like seeing is often taken for granted. Until I began to lose my hearing, I took it for granted.

This book is written to help the millions of folks who have lost some or all of their hearing. Some are hearing-impaired, others are deaf.

My goal is to present information for the average consumer who is dealing with this problem. The book presents a common-sense approach to finding some winning solutions that work.

No one ever said that there is one simple answer. In life, we have to develop strategies that allow us to function in this world, in spite of loss.

This book is designed to educate and lighten the load of the hearing-impaired. Hopefully, in this bionic age, future winning solutions will help conquer hearing loss.

ACKNOWLEDGEMENTS

My thanks to my family, my friends, and my loyal students. Their loyalty has allowed me to rise above loss, and help others do the same.

My thanks go to the book buyers who were kind enough to read and comment upon this book.

This book would not have been possible without the support that I have received from professionals in the field who have been kind enough to share new research and information.

My professional interviews have included many audiologists in both Rhode Island and Florida. Also, I have had contact with doctors at Massachusetts Eye and Ear Infirmary, John Hopkins Hospital, Jackson Memorial Hospital, and Rhode Island Hospital.

My research also includes contacts with manufacturers who produce the latest devices to help people with hearing impairment.

Every effort has been made to obtain permission for each reference,but general information is as accurate as possible.

It is important for the reader to refer to the Notice to the Reader that follows this page.

NOTICE TO THE READER

SINCE HEARING PROBLEMS VARY, READERS ARE ADVISED TO SEEK PROFESSIONAL HELP FROM A LICENSED PHYSICIAN.

This book is a guide to information and support for the consumer. The book will help to explain some simple solutions to a serious problem.

DISCLAIMER

The book should be used to supplement information. It should not replace any medical advice, and the author will not assume any responsibility for information that may change.

The reader must follow the advice of the physician and the professionals in the field.

The author is a hearing-impaired educator. She is a Professor Emerita, and has taught at six different colleges. She also runs THE WRITING WORKSHOP in Naples, Florida. She divides her time between Florida and Rhode Island.

viii

CHAPTER ONE

DEFINING THE PROBLEM

Hearing loss affects millions of people of all ages. It is one of the most common handicapping conditions. Yet, it is often misunderstood.

Basically, hearing loss is a reduction of a person's ability to hear. Since the loss is invisible, it is not obvious. An estimated one third of the population over 65 is hearing-impaired. By age 75, one half of the population is affected.

Children can also be affected. Indeed, a baby can be born deaf. The problem is universal. If you live to a ripe old age, the odds are that you will develop a hearing problem.

Age-related hearing loss has a technical name, prebycusis. Prebycusis is caused by changes in the hair cells in the cochlea in the ear. Studies have shown that as we age, we lose nerve cells in the internal part of the ear.

There are different types of hearing loss. The first type is called a conductive hearing loss. In this case there is a problem with the transfer of sound to the inner ear. The cause could be infection, earwax, or damage to the eardrum.

The second type is called sensorineural hearing loss. It is caused by damage to the cells in the inner ear or the nerve itself, or a combination of both. Generally, this type of loss cannot be reversed.

A third type of loss is called a central hearing loss. In this case there could be a tumor causing the loss, or damage to the central nervous system. For example, a person who has had a stroke could have this type of loss.

Some people have a combination of any one or more of these problems. It is important to visit an ear doctor to get a correct diagnosis. The physician will have an audiologist give you hearing tests to discover the extent of the loss.

The physician might order other medical tests if the loss is severe. Visit a doctor early to get the correct diagnosis and begin rehabilitation.

Hearing problems are not simple. People try to ignore or hide the symptoms. There are many signs that are signals:

1. Pain
2. Dizziness
3. Ringing in the ears
4. Hearing loss
5. Drainage from the ear
6. Speech deterioration

Naturally, if a person fails to respond appropriately to sound, one needs to assess the reason. Is it because they are unable to hear, or is it for a different reason? This failure to respond could signal there are problems.

Defining the problem includes noting if the loss is mild, moderate, severe, or profound. Is the loss in one ear or both ears? How severe is the loss? An analysis is needed to differentiate the type of loss.

By seeking the appropriate medical help early, corrective therapy can begin. If you are unsure about the diagnosis, think about getting a second or third opinion. Select professionals from different locations, and then compare what each one says. Finding accurate information can take time, but it is time well-spent. Hearing is important, and you want to follow the most logical corrective procedures.

SOLUTIONS FROM CHAPTER ONE

- ADMIT YOU HAVE A PROBLEM.

- GET AN ACCURATE DIAGNOSIS FROM A PHYSICIAN.

- MAKE SURE THERE ARE NO TUMORS CAUSING HEARING LOSS.

- DISCUSS YOUR OPTIONS WITH QUALIFIED PROFESSIONALS.

- EARLY INTERVENTION MAKES SENSE.

- GET TESTED BY AN AUDIOLOGIST.

- SELECT PROFESSIONALS YOU CAN TRUST.

- GET A SECOND OPINION.

- INTERVIEW THE PROFESSIONALS YOU SELECT.

- CHOOSE AN AUDIOLOGIST THAT CARES AND WILL GIVE YOU EXTRA TIME AS NEEDED.

- IF POSSIBLE, FIND PROFESSIONALS THAT ARE CONVENIENT. YOU WILL BE MAKING MORE THAN ONE VISIT.

CHAPTER TWO

EMOTIONAL REACTIONS TO HEARING LOSS

The emotional reactions to hearing loss are tremendous. Just admitting that you have a problem hearing is the beginning of the solution. Initially one can feel frustration, anger, resentment, rejection, sadness, awkwardness, isolation, and embarrassment. To come to terms with hearing loss you must admit to yourself and others that you have a problem. Now you can take the next step and find some acceptable solutions.

There are many products on the market that will help you, and these will be discussed in depth in other parts of the book. This chapter will focus on simple things you can do to improve your emotional attitude.

PHYSICAL EXERCISE

Physical exercise is a wonderful stress-reducer. Daily exercise makes sense. It will help to improve your mind as well as your body. Think about doing your exercise in the morning. This way you are charging up your metabolism right from the start of the day.

Morning exercise also helps you to handle the stress and problems that take place throughout the day. It will act as a daily reminder that you have to start out each day with a positive approach to what will take place. Even if you are working, try to get up earlier to do your exercise.

Walking is an excellent choice for most of us. You do not need any special equipment, and you can do it with friends or by yourself. It is highly aerobic, and you can vary where you walk so that you will not get bored.

The pace and intensity of your walks can also vary based on your level of fitness. Using good posture, walking can be faster as time goes on. Keep your head up, swing your arms, and take deep breaths as you walk. You will be adding oxygen to your body, and stress relief to your mind. Walking will help your heart, your lungs, your flexibility, and most important your attitude. As you begin to enjoy the walk, your body and mind will relax. Suddenly you will notice scenery that you never saw. Pick a pretty area and begin to appreciate the natural beauty that surrounds you. Mother nature has many wonders for us to enjoy. We need to take the time to notice.

Swimming is another excellent cardiovascular sport. If you have arthritis, swimming puts no stress on your joints. It can be done indoors or outdoors, and you can adjust the length of your swim as well as the pace. Do use protection for your swim. Buy earplugs and swim eyeglasses. After each swim shower. This will wash off the chlorine. Even after an ocean swim do not forget to shower.

Other fun sports include: tennis, golf, dancing, bicycling, and any activity that gets you moving. The body is meant to be used. Vary your sports so that you do not stress just one part of the body. It is healthy to try new sports so you have more choices. If one part of the body is sore, do an activity that is easier. The Greeks were not wrong when they said, "A sound mind in a sound body."

THERAPEUTIC MASSAGE

Another great stress-reducer is therapeutic massage. There is no doubt that massage is an antidote to stress. On the physical side massage helps with circulation. It reduces muscle tension, and it nourishes the skin. If you have strained a part of the body, massage can help to heal the area. Massage feels so good, and it is also an emotional healer. There are different types of massages, and you should discuss with the massage therapist what will work best for you. Interview the therapist, and work with someone you can talk with easily. Massage can be done at home or in an office. Schedule your massage when you are not going to be rushed. In this way you will get the full benefit.

MEDITATION

Meditation is a relaxation technique that operates in the realm of mind/body medicine. It is a way to gain relief from stress. By focusing the mind on peaceful thoughts, the body begins to relax. Buddhist monks have used this technique for years. Today medical doctors are realizing that it makes sense. To learn meditation you can use audiotapes, videotapes, take classes, and work with instructors. Regardless of the approach, the result will help you learn how to relax. You will feel better, and coping with stress will get easier.

HUMOR

Everyone enjoys a good laugh. It is healthy for you. With hearing problems you will not always understand what people are saying. Try not to get too concerned. If you make a mistake, laugh at yourself. Let the error go, and do not get bent out of shape. Most errors can be corrected. Many of the things that upset us really are not that important. Accept the fact that this will happen, and move on.

POSITIVE MENTAL ATTITUDE

As you begin each day you have choices. It is much healthier to maintain a positive attitude. No one enjoys loss of any kind, but it happens. There is a saying, "Laugh and the world laughs with you, cry and you cry alone." How true this is. Forget you have problems, concentrate on what you can do, don't worry about what you did not hear. If it is really important you can discover the facts at a different time. Most things are of minor importance. Indeed, sometimes it is a blessing not to hear certain information. If you are unaware of certain problems, you may be better off and worry less.

DIET

You are what you eat. Your body needs nutrition, and you have to make choices to stay healthy. Drink plenty of water. It is not fattening, and six to eight glasses each day will help with weight control and hydration. Eat a variety of foods and eat mostly fruits and vegetables. Try to cut out the sweets, and substitute healthy snacks like carrot sticks and celery. Add skim milk, yogurt, and low fat cheese, and this will help with calcium. Talk with a nutritionist about what you should be eating. When you eat the right kinds of food, you will look better and feel better.

KEEP YOUR LIFE SIMPLE

Keep your life simple. Life is easier that way. When things get too complicated, it is tough emotionally. Take naps, and do not try to do everything in one day. Allow enough time to relax and enjoy the ride. In the long run you will feel better, and you will accomplish more if you slow down and relax.

Learn to arrange your day based on what is most important. Sometimes you will have to make last minute changes. Be flexible and if you have to adjust your schedule, try not to get bent out of shape. Get help with your projects when you need to. Try to include others in your life, and call upon them as needed. People like to help, and it makes them feel good when they are needed. As long as your needs are within reason and in a time frame that works for others, you will be able to share and lighten your day. It is important that you show appreciation. People do like to know that their efforts are noticed. Saying thank you does make good sense.

SOLUTIONS FROM CHAPTER TWO

- YOUR EMOTIONS WILL BE AFFECTED.
- TRY PHYSICAL EXERCISE FOR STRESS RELIEF.
- WALKING IS AN EXCELLENT EXERCISE.
- SWIMMING AND FUN SPORTS PERK UP YOUR ATTITUDE.
- ENJOY A MASSAGE.
- MEDITATION IS A RELAXATION TECHNIQUE.
- MAINTAIN A SENSE OF HUMOR.
- LEARN TO LAUGH AT YOURSELF.
- DRINK PLENTY OF WATER.
- TALK WITH A NUTRITIONIST ABOUT A HEALTHY DIET.
- KEEP YOUR LIFE SIMPLE.
- TAKE NAPS AND ENJOY YOURSELF.

CHAPTER THREE

CHILDREN AND HEARING LOSS

It is well-documented that almost any of the childhood infections can affect hearing in children. Also, heredity may cause deafness as well. There are about 400 different types of genetic hearing problems. Some occur at birth, others can occur later in life. New research has found several genes linked to deafness.

Children with hearing problems can be born to parents with normal hearing. Scientists have discovered that a gene plays a significant role in the development of the cells essential to hearing. This gene sends a signal to ear cells to mature into hair cells in the inner ear. Hair cells are responsible for both hearing and balance. If these cells do not develop, or if they are destroyed, they do not regenerate.

In addition, many diseases can be passed down from the mother to the fetus. For example, if the mother has German measles during pregnancy, this disease can cause birth defects in the child's hearing. Likewise premature birth, mumps, scarlet fever, all the diseases that a mother could have during the pregnancy can affect the hearing of the child.

As a result it is important for the mother to have the infant tested as early as possible to detect hearing loss. After all, children learn speech patterns through hearing and imitation. Any problems need to be addressed as early as possible. If undetected, hearing loss leads to major social and academic complications.

Infants can be fitted with hearing devices as young as four weeks old. Currently there is legislation before Congress to mandate universal newborn screening. It is done in 34 states already. The earlier hearing loss is diagnosed, the better it will be for the child. Presently the American Academy of Pediatrics recommends that all newborns be checked for hearing ability. Once the child has been diagnosed with a hearing problem, devices can be added to help with speech development.

In addition to hearing aids, FM systems are the most common assistive listening devices used with children. By using an FM listening system, a child will be able to hear the teacher's voice regardless of the distance between the child and the teacher.

Many school districts employ certified audiologists who specialize in educational settings. They work with the teacher to determine the best plan for the child's education.

It is important to work with both an audiologist and an early intervention team to evaluate the best program for the child. If a child is deaf, then different schools and plans exist. Most members of the deaf culture use American Sign Language, and this is a separate educational program.

The Individuals with Disabilities Education Act ensures that children who have hearing loss receive free programs from birth to age 3, and throughout the school years as well. Early intervention programs involve multidisciplinary services. The goal is to enhance the family's understanding of the child's needs and build a support system to monitor the child's progress.

In a separate chapter, the subject of cochlear implants will be covered. This is another possibility for the deaf child. For more information on children and hearing loss, parents can contact the American Speech, Language , and Hearing Association for additional advice. Their phone number is 1-800-638-8255.

The lack of early detection of hearing problems in children is one of the major health problems today. Educating the mother before the child is born is essential. A woman must learn how to care for herself before pregnancy so that the chances of having a healthy baby will be greater. The mother is the key, and her health habits will directly influence what happens to the baby. She must take on the responsibility of learning as much as she can to help the odds of producing a healthy child.

SOLUTIONS FROM CHAPTER THREE

- HEARING LOSS CAN BE GENETIC.

- EDUCATING MOTHERS BEFORE PREGNANCY MAKES SENSE.

- NEWBORN SCREENING CAN BE DONE.

- PRENATAL DISEASES CAN BE PREVENTED.

- PREGNANT WOMEN MUST AVOID SMOKING AND ALCOHOL TO PROTECT THE FETUS.

- A QUALIFIED TEAM APPROACH CAN HELP CHILDREN SUCCEED.

- CHILDREN CAN BE FITTED WITH HEARING AIDS.

- CHILDREN CAN HAVE COCHLEAR IMPLANTS.

- CHILDREN CAN USE ASSISTIVE LISTENING DEVICES.

- CHILDREN NEED A STRONG SUPPORT SYSTEM.

- CHILDREN ARE ENTITLED TO SPECIAL SCHOOL SERVICES.

CHAPTER FOUR

BUYING HEARING AIDS

Buying hearing aids can be confusing and costly. To simplify the process, analyze your needs and your budget. To begin, confirm that you need hearing aids. A qualified physician will do an exam. An audiologist will do a hearing test. If the test results show the need, the doctor will then sign a certificate of need.

There is no hearing aid that will give you back your hearing. The aid will increase your awareness of sounds. It is important to realize that hearing aids will not restore normal hearing. What you can do is sample different hearing aid products. Hearing aids come in different styles and sizes. There are small products that go into the ear and can hardly be seen. Other aids fit right in the ear, and then there are products that go behind the ear. For a greater loss of hearing the behind-the-ear product works best. This model is attached to an earmold, and because it is a bit larger, it can hold more microphones. Also, if the product needs adjustment, by removing the earmold, you can send it for repair. Usually, the same earmold can be attached to a loaner or a different hearing aid. Many companies will lend you a replacement while your product is being fixed. It pays to ask before you purchase your model what they will do for you in case of repair problems.

A hearing aid is like a pair of shoes. It must fit and be comfortable. The smaller less visible aids are going to be more expensive, and more difficult to insert. In buying a hearing aid you need to be practical. What product will work, will be comfortable to wear, and will give you the greatest clarity? The smallest products may be less visible, but they are easiest to lose, and sometimes hardest to insert. Also, they are not appropriate for every hearing loss.

Hearing aids come in different materials. For people with sensitive skin, they have earmolds and aids that are hypoallergenic. Even though the product is labeled allergy free, this does not insure it will work for all users. It is possible to request that the earmold be boiled to remove any plastic residue. In extreme cases, hearing aids can even be implanted. Generally, most people can find an available product that will work.

Hearing aids are sold by dealers and audiologists. The audiologist has more knowledge and training. The dealer

18

may be licensed, but this does not compare to the education that the audiologist has received. It is wise to interview several audiologists to see if you could work with them. Buying a hearing aid will require more than one visit. Adjustments and repairs mean that you will have an extended relationship with your supplier. Consider finding an audiologist who is pleasant, gives you time, and is convenient. Above all ask to see the purchase contract from each audiologist that you interview. Payment terms vary, and even though they may tell you that you have a free trial period, the terms are misleading. The trial period varies, and can be extended upon mutual agreement. The cost of the trial is not free. If an earmold is required this is not free. Sometimes they add on a service charge if you decide not to keep the product.

Today there has been an explosion in the number of digital hearing aids on the market. Are the digital hearing aids really superior to their analog counterparts? To determine whether they work better for you, try them, and also try the less expensive older analog products. The older models have dials you can control for volume without running to the audiologist. Not all digital models can be adjusted without an audiologist. This could be a nuisance. Since trying different products requires time, there may be a service charge.

We normally hear with two ears. Most people should consider getting two hearing aids. Some may even need an emergency set. Most dispensers will give you a loaner in the event that your hearing aids need repair. With an earmold

19

this is simple, and your earmold slips on to the new product.

Take the time to sample different hearing aid products. Only by trying them will you discover what works best for you. Buying a hearing aid is a bit like purchasing a diamond. You need to trust your dealer, you need to shop and compare prices, and you need to be comfortable with the product. You should pay by credit card, and ask if the payment can be divided so you do not pay at all once. If you are a senior citizen, ask for a senior discount. Also ask if any hearing aid companies are offering any special promotions. It does make sense to ask these questions.

For people who do not want to make a major investment you can even purchase a disposable hearing aid. Disposable aids come in different sizes, and generally the newer models are about $79 for two months. No battery is required, and at the end of the two months, the product no longer works. They do have different strengths as well, but the earmold only comes in three sizes. You will see if you even like a hearing aid, but this type is not fitted to you, and may not stay in the ear as required. It is tough to get the exact fit. A disposable aid will give you a sense of what it is like to wear a hearing aid, but the custom-made more expensive models are far more effective.

Fitted hearing aids are much more costly. Prices usually begin around $1000 and can go as high as $4000 for each ear. Once you decide what you want, consider buying the extended warranty. For about $30 each year, this will insure the product, and in case of loss or theft, you will get a new one. Most insurance plans will not cover hearing aids. Also, the cost of hearing aids is not covered by Medicare. Unless you are a veteran, with a war-related hearing loss, you will pay the bill. It is, however, a medical expense, and you can check with your accountant to see if you are entitled to a tax deduction.

Hearing aids are meant to improve ease of communication. They are not new ears. You need to have realistic expectations. Time is required to adjust to the new sounds you will be hearing. Be patient with yourself and maintain a positive attitude. They will improve your communication. Once you get used to wearing them, they will be part of your daily attire. Hearing aids do not restore hearing to normal like eyeglasses do for vision, but they can improve your hearing and listening ability, and they can substantially improve the quality of your life.

Finally, beware of mail-order hearing-aid sales. You will need an audiologist because follow-up care is required. You may save a small amount of money, but you need the added support of professional help, and this is not always available when buying online.

SOLUTIONS FROM CHAPTER FOUR

- MAKE SURE YOU NEED THE PRODUCT.

- HAVE AN AUDIOLOGICAL EVALUATION.

- INTERVIEW SEVERAL AUDIOLOGISTS.

- DO NOT BUY WITHOUT A TRIAL PERIOD.

- FIND OUT THE TIME LINES AND PRICE FOR A TRIAL.

- SMALLER HEARING AIDS WILL COST MORE MONEY.

- FOR A GREATER HEARING LOSS BEHIND-THE-EAR MODELS GIVE YOU MORE POWER.

- YOU DO NOT ALWAYS NEED THE MOST EXPENSIVE PRODUCT.

- ASK TO SEE THE PURCHASE CONTRACT.

- FIND OUT ABOUT PAYMENT OPTIONS.

- COMPARE PRICES AT SEVERAL PLACES.

- AVOID ONLINE SALES.

- FIND OUT ABOUT LOANERS IN CASE OF REPAIRS.

- TRY ONE AND TWO AIDS TO SEE WHAT WORKS BEST.

- CONSIDER A CONVIENT LOCATION FOR YOUR PROFESSIONALS.

- BUYING HEARING AIDS REQUIRES MORE THAN ONE VISIT SO TAKE YOUR TIME.

- CONSIDER LESS EXPENSIVE PRODUCTS. THEY MAY DO THE JOB FOR YOU.

- DO NOT SIGN ANY CONTRACT DURING THE TRIAL PERIOD.

- SHOP FOR THE BEST PRICE.

- DISCUSS THE LENGTH OF THE TRIAL PERIOD.

- COMPARE PRICES AND SERVICES.

- FIND OUT THE TERMS OF THE WARRANTY.

- LEARN ABOUT THE EXTENDED WARRANTY.

- MOST HOME INSURANCE POLICIES DO NOT COVER HEARING AIDS.

- KEEP A RECORD OF YOUR COSTS FOR HEARING AIDS. SUBMIT THE BILLS TO YOUR ACCOUNTANT. THE PRODUCTS ARE A MEDICAL EXPENSE.

- IF YOU ARE A VETERAN YOU MAY APPLY FOR VETERAN'S BENEFITS.

- BEWARE OF DECEPTIVE ADS.

- AVOID HIGH-POWERED SALES PEOPLE.

- TAKE YOUR TIME AND DO RESEARCH ON PRICES AND PRODUCTS.

- CONSIDER TWO HEARING AIDS FOR BETTER RESULTS.

24

CHAPTER FIVE

ASSISTIVE TECHNOLOGIES

What are assistive listening devices? An assistive device is any type of equipment that can help you function better in communications situations. Examples of devices include: amplified telephones, television aids, alerting devices, and even trained dogs.

TELEPHONES

Telephone aids are often a necessity. The telephone is one of the biggest obstacles to communication. Part of the problem is that you have no visual cues. If you are unable to see the person, it is hard to know what they are saying.

You can get an amplified phone. Also, you can have

Caller ID. Both these devices do help. You can also have a telecoil switch put on your hearing aid. The telecoil also called the T-switch allows you to hear without feedback from the phone line.

There are also text telephones, and they allow you to type a message over the telephone network. Today, by dialing 711, you can be connected to a relay operator who will receive and relay your message. She will then type the response back to you. Relay operators are working 24 hours a day. There is no additional charge for local calls. There are also special long distance rates. You need to contact your telephone carrier for the details.

The use of the text telephone does require some education. You need to learn the correct procedures to make it work. You can call the relay operator at 711 for help. Also, most of the phone companies have a special department for customers with disabilities. Ask the business office to connect you to the correct department.

Amplified phones are also available. You need to find out if they are compatible with your hearing aids. Newer phones now require this feature. If your hearing aid has the T- switch, this should eliminate the screaming noise called feedback.

In certain states you can receive a free phone that is loaned to you. Ask your doctor or your audiologist how to get this equipment. There is a form that they will give you, that they must sign. This form confirms your hearing loss. In case you need more information, have the doctor or hearing professional write out the instructions for you. The free phones vary depending on the extent of your loss. There are amplified phones as well as text telephones available. You need to specify the extent of your loss. Have the professional list the type of phone that will be best for your needs.

For travel purposes, you can even buy a portable amplifier that will attach to the headset of any phone. This is handy in case you are in a location that does not have an amplified phone.

The various types of equipment can be purchased through catalogues, online, and through your hearing professionals. At the end of this chapter there is a list of companies that carry these products. Most of the companies will send you a free catalogue. You can contact them by phone, or by going online to their website. Most of them have an e-mail address. By searching on the computer you will discover additional information about the various products

When you are researching the products, it does pay to compare prices and warranties. When you buy a product use your credit card. This will protect you in case there are any problems.

TELEVISION

Today new televisions are required to have a closed-captioned feature. Like foreign films, the dialogue is written as it is spoken. This allows you to read what the speakers are saying. You can also follow the dialogue. By watching, reading, and listening, you will begin to comprehend.

Another aid is called Direct Ear. This device uses wireless audio technology and invisible infrared-light-waves to carry the sound directly to a set of earphones that you wear. You can use these earphones with or without your hearing aids. The listener can adjust the volume by using a separate volume control under the chin, and others can watch the program at a comfortable level for them. The headset can also be used in theaters that are equipped with infrared-light. You need to inquire before attending a performance what type of equipment is available for the hearing-impaired.

FM LISTENING SYSTEMS

Personal FM systems are another listening device. The system is like a miniature radio station. There is a transmitter microphone used by the speaker, and a receiver used by the listener. The FCC has assigned frequencies for use by public and private systems.

FM systems are very useful in a classroom. The teacher

can speak directly to the student thereby eliminating background noise. The sound is carried through the air, and the receiver can wear the system with or without a hearing aid. Each student needs a separate device for direct input to take place.

ALERTING DEVICES

There are many alerting devices that send signals by light, sound, and vibration. For example you can purchase an extra-loud-alarm clock, and some clocks have an attachment that vibrates the bed to wake you. Also, there are doorbells that have signals that are visual. Some connect to a lamp that lights when the bell rings.

Visual alarms are also available for driving. Your car can be equipped to alert you to sirens, as well as to turn signals. You need to ask the service department about special equipment. Very bright strobe lights are often used for smoke alarms or if the phone rings. Modern technology has come up with many helpful aids for the hearing-impaired.

WALKING CANES

A colorful cane is also a safety device. When crossing the street the driver is not aware that you have a hearing problem. By using a colorful cane, the driver can see that you may need extra time crossing the street. Canes can be designed to coordinate with your outfit. By contacting Nshu4@aol.com you can order a cane designed with you in mind. Learn to use a cane as a signal to drivers that you need extra time to cross the street. When the drivers see you have a problem, they will be more cautious.

HEARING DOGS

Hearing-ear-dogs can be any breed or size. They are specially trained and many states have training programs. Listed below are some national programs that exist. You need to contact your state to discover if a similar program exists. Normally there is a waiting list. Contact your local SPCA to find out the details.

American Humane Association
PO Box 1266
Denver, CO 80231
303-695-0811

Canine Companions for Independence
PO Box 446
Santa Rosa, CA 95402

Canine Helpers for the Handicapped
5705 Ridge Road
Lockport, NY 14904
716-433-4035

Dogs for the Deaf
110175 Wheeler Rd.
Central Point, OR 97502
503-899-7177

National Hearing Dog Center
1116 S. Main
Athol, MA 01331
508-249-9264

Red Acre Farm Hearing Dog Center
109 Red Acre Road
Stow MA 01775
508-897-5370

Listed below are some of the names and phone numbers of the companies that sell the devices and the technology mentioned in this chapter.

- American Communications Corp. 800-203-3491
- AT&T National Speech Needs Center 800-233-1222
- Audio Enhancement 314-367-6141
- G.N. Donavon 800-247-5343
- General Technologies 916-962-9225
- Harris Communications 800-825-9187
- Hear You Are 201-347-7662
- Nationwide Flashing Signals 301-589-6671
- Radio Shack. Check for your local listing.
- Sennheiser 302-434-9190
- Siemens Hearing Instruments 908-562-6600
- Sonic Alert 313-656-3110

This list does not endorse any particular business. There are many additional companies that offer hearing products. By going online, you can search other sources. Most of the businesses will send you a free catalogue. Prices and warranties on products will vary. Ask for discounts or discontinued products. Certain items may be on sale. It never hurts to ask. By doing some research you can save both time and money.

INTERPRETERS

Since the 1960's federal and state laws have been enacted regarding interpreters for the deaf and hearing-impaired. Oral interpreters are trained to silently mouth a speaker's words. They have special training and certification. By calling your local Office of Vocational Rehabilitation of your local hearing center, you can find out the details. A person who is hearing-impaired can request an interpreter who is provided free of charge to agencies that receive federal funds. In addition, the Education for Handicapped Children Act of 1975 requires that services of an interpreter must be written into a student's educational plan. The services are paid for by the school system. Most states also pay for an interpreter in the civil and federal courts. Check with your state governor's office to connect with the appropriate agency.

SIGN LANGUAGE INTERPRETERS

A sign language interpreter is a person skilled in the ability to translate the meaning of spoken words into sign language. There are various forms of sign language. In the United States we use American Sign Language. Other countries have different sign languages. There is no one universal sign language.

There are variations in sign language just as there are variations in spoken language from different regions. The signs can vary based upon different locations. ASL is the abbreviation used for American Sign Language. It has been accepted as a complete language. Just as it takes practice to learn a foreign language, sign language requires education and practice as well. In the United States, ASL is an integral part of deaf culture. There are numerous online sites that exist with links for additional information. Three web addresses are listed below:

1. Deaf World Web:dww.deafworldweb.org
2. Registry of Interpreters for the Deaf
   Web: www.rad.org
3. National Information Center on Deafness
   Web: www.gallaudet.edu/-nicd

33

SOLUTIONS FROM CHAPTER FIVE

- AMPLIFIED TELEPHONES.
- CALLER ID.
- TEXT TELEPHONES.
- RELAY OPERATORS.
- PORTABLE TELEPHONE ATTACHMENTS FOR TRAVEL.
- CLOSED-CAPTIONED TELEVISION.
- DIRECT EAR INFRARED HEADPHONES.
- PERSONAL FM LISTENING SYSTEMS.
- ALERTING SYSTEMS.
- EXTRA-LOUD-ALARM CLOCKS.
- CLOCKS WITH VIBRATING ATTACHMENTS.
- HEARING DOGS.
- DECORATIVE WALKING CANES.
- HEARING AIDS.
- INTERPRETERS.
- AUTOMATIC LIGHT SIGNALERS.
- TELECOIL SWITCHES IN HEARING AIDS.

CHAPTER SIX

STRATEGIES THAT WORK

There are many strategies that work for hearing loss. As you try the different techniques, you may discover which ones you like the best. In addition, add some of your own that are not included. You may learn from others who also have the same problems.

PACING YOUR ACITIVITIES: Give yourself a break. Try to allow extra time for each task. Realize that most things will take longer than you expected. You will handle things more smoothly with extra time. If you have time in your favor, you will be less likely to panic and get stressed. When you are in control of a situation, you will be more relaxed. You will also be able to consider alternatives based on the situation. By jamming your schedule, you force yourself to rush. The old saying, "Haste makes waste" is true. Spread out your errands, and in the long run, they will get done without tension. Everything does not have to be done in the same day.

LIFE HAS BUMPS IN THE ROAD. Going more slowly cushions unexpected change. Try to schedule one thing at a time. Often things do occur that you cannot control. Road construction, accidents, and bad weather, these are some of the problems that you face when driving. Delays in travel go beyond your control. Most things are not an emergency. Take some extra time en route, and you will feel better when you arrive at your destination.

SMALL GROUPS MAKES SENSE: Given a choice, it is much easier to hear in a small group. A large group means many cross-conversations. Even when you have good hearing, it is difficult to concentrate when there is a large crowd of people. Face the person you need to address. Watching them helps in many ways. You can read their lips and their gestures. Tell the people that you are hard of hearing, and ask them speak slowly and with good volume. Request that they do not put their hands over their mouth so that you can read their lips. Body gestures help to support ideas. Perhaps at meetings, you can request that a group secretary be appointed so that you and others can have notes to review. Being able to read what has been said is good for you, and others will appreciate it as well.

PRIOR INFORMATION HELPS: Keep informed on the subjects you and others need to discuss. Research is essential to being informed. By doing advance work, you will be better able to communicate your ideas. Try to use the internet and the newspaper to keep informed on news. Generally, it is much easier to understand a conversation when you have prior information on the subject matter. You might contact a group leader before a meeting to see the agenda. That way if you do not understand an issue, you can discuss it before the meeting. Also, notify the leader that you do have hearing problems. Perhaps you could be seated so that you could see clearly and hear to the best of your ability. In a classroom consider sitting in the front row. This way you will be closer to the teacher.

CALLER ID: As stated previously, advance information helps. If you know who is calling when you pick up the receiver, you will not struggle with voice identification. This makes the call easier for you. Even with prior information, the phone can be a problem. The caller is invisible, so you are unable to read lips and gestures. Try to have an amplified phone available. If needed you can purchase a small portable device that you can carry with you for travel. In the event there is no amplified phone, use your own attachment as needed.

GOOD LIGHTING: If you can see someone easily, you can notice gestures. Also, try to read their lips as well.

Position yourself so that the light shines on the speaker. This will help you see facial expressions easily. Consider carrying a small flashlight. At night this will help you make your way when it is dark. Many streets are not well-lit, and often street lights are limited or just don't work. Even with good hearing, it makes sense to carry a flashlight. Sidewalks are uneven and can be dangerous. If you have light it is much easier to navigate.

CARPETING, CURTAINS, AND AN ACCOUSTICAL CEILING: The environment in restaurants and public rooms does make a difference. Whenever possible ask for a quiet table in a restaurant. Tell the host or hostess you have a hearing problem. You can even call in advance and make a reservation stating your problem. Usually they will try to help you out.

USE ASSISTIVE EQUIPMENT: There are many products that you can purchase to enhance sounds. See Chapter Five for the details. Become familiar with the different types of equipment. Today you can request equipment at most theaters and places of worship. Ask the manager at the theater what devices they carry for the hard-of-hearing. Federal programs mandate that provisions be made for people with hearing problems.

LIP READING: Courses exist that can train you to read lips. Check with the senior agencies as well as the local colleges to find a course. Also, contact your state government, and they can refer you to the agency that handles disabilites. Lip reading is a skill. You need to take a course to learn how to do it. It takes education and practice. Since it can help a great deal in communication, it is worth the time to learn how to do it.

INTERNET AND E-MAIL MAKE SENSE: Since you can read messages on the internet, it makes good sense to use it. Not only does it save time, but it also saves money. There are travel bargains, and you can connect all over the world for the price of your online server. Even if you do not own a computer, you can go to the library and the equipment there is free of charge. In addition, you can rent a computer, and some banks and coffee houses offer free computer services. It does pay to learn how to use this valuable tool. Consider hiring a tutor. Many high school students are very capable and would love to earn some money teaching this skill.

WRITING JOURNAL: Keep a writing journal. List what works and add things that make you happy. Try to focus on positive things. Use whatever system works for you. Even if you have to use a pencil and paper to understand, do it. If you were travelling in a foreign country, you would use a variety of resources to communicate. Learning to live with hearing loss is like learning a new language. You would not be shy in another country, so apply the same rules. People will accept you as you accept yourself. The rule of thumb is to try until things work for you. Do not isolate yourself. Be optimistic, have a sense of humor, and others will respond. As the saying goes, JUST DO IT!

CREATIVITY: Try whatever system works for you. Pretend that you have now invented a new language. You may only hear half of what people say, but by being creative you can try to understand the full message. Use clues and main ideas to help you. Ask people to repeat ideas that are important. Write out things that are very important, and check yourself for accuracy. Creativity counts, make it work for you.

SOLUTIONS FROM CHAPTER SIX

- PACE YOURSELF ALLOW EXTRA TIME FOR EACH TASK.

- SMALL GROUPS MAKE SENSE.

- FACE THE PERSON WHEN YOU TALK.

- EXPLAIN THAT YOU MUST SEE THEIR FACE WHEN THEY TALK. VISIBILITY COUNTS AND MAKES IT EASIER TO READ LIPS.

- GET PRIOR INFORMATION ON SUBJECT MATTER TO AID UNDERSTANDING.

- GOOD LIGHTING HELPS TO READ LIPS.

- SELECT A QUIET CORNER IN RESTAURNTS.

- TELL THE HOST OR HOSTESS IN RESTAURANTS THAT YOU HAVE A HEARING PROBLEM. REQUEST A QUIET TABLE.

- USE THE INTERNET FOR APPOINTMENTS AND COMMUNICATIONS WITH FAMILY AND FRIENDS.

- E-MAIL INFORMATION FOR BUSINESS. YOU CAN KEEP A COPY FOR YOUR RECORDS.

- KEEP A WRITING JOURNAL. LIST WHAT TECHNIQUES WORK FOR YOU. LIST PROBLEM AREAS. TRY TO ELIMINATE WHAT AREAS CREATE A PROBLEM. SEEK NEW SOLUTIONS FOR PRIOR PROBLEMS.

- FOCUS ON POSITIVE THINGS THAT MAKE YOU HAPPY.

- GET PLENTY OF REST. TAKE NAPS TO REFRESH YOURSELF.

CHAPTER SEVEN

THE COMPUTER, E-MAIL, THE INTERNET

One of the most valuable tools to assist the hearing-impaired is the computer. Not only does the computer open up the world, but it also saves time and money. Best of all, no hearing skills are required. One simply needs to read the text, and follow computer directions. Using the computer will give you access to the internet and e-mail. Both are extremely valuable.

Learning to use the computer does require training. A few lessons will definitely help. There are many classes available, but even more beneficial are private lessons. If possible, a capable teenager makes a good tutor. You should compare prices for lessons, and you do need a teacher who can sit next to you and be patient. Even with lessons, it does take practice.

Using e-mail will allow you to keep in touch with friends and family. By paying a small monthly fee to an online service provider, you will be able to send messages all over the world. It is best to research the different rates that the online providers offer. Compare rates and learn which company will give you the best deal. It may take several phone calls, but find out the different plans that are offered. Sometimes a limited plan will be cheaper, and it may give you enough time online to accomplish what you need. If you are a senior, request a senior rate. If you belong to AARP there is a discount.

Many service providers will allow you to try their service free of charge for a short period of time. Today you can even get cable service to connect directly online. Otherwise,you will be using your phone line to connect with your internet provider. Ask your friends and family which service provider they use, and you can learn from others what works best before you sign up.

Like any tool, one must use common sense. Messages on the web are not totally private, so you must use caution. Be careful with any online buying as well. Make sure the companies that you select have some type of protection in case you need to use your credit card. Once you have signed with a company you will receive many e-mails from all types of companies. These unsolicited ads can be ignored, and you need not respond. Indeed, you will learn to delete them, since most of the messages are just ads for business.

The rewards with the computer far outweigh the risks. What a great way to save time and energy. In addition, the internet is great for research. You can select any category, and by pushing the appropriate button you will find out new infomation on any subject. You can even do a search on any subject and you will be amazed at the vast amount of information that you can select. Most of the information is current, but you need to be selective for accuracy. Research from the company that produces a product could be biased.

When you decide to own your own computer, you will have many choices. Do you want a laptop that is light and portable, or would you prefer a larger computer? Look at the various models and talk to the sales personnel to learn about the different models. At first it may be confusing, but perservere. The prices for computers have come down, and by checking the newpaper there are always sales. Again, seniors should ask for discounts. You will not get the discount without making a request.

Learning the computer requires time and tenacity. Today all the schools teach students computer skills. Since the world is now operating on computer systems, it becomes essential for employment that you learn these skills. There is always something new to learn, but hang in there, do not give up. It is definitely worth the time and effort.

SOLUTIONS FROM CHAPTER SEVEN

- COMPUTERS REQUIRE NO HEARING SKILLS.
- COMPUTERS LET YOU CONNECT EASILY.
- E-MAIL LETS YOU KEEP IN TOUCH.
- E-MAIL SAVES MONEY ON LONG-DISTANCE CALLS.
- E-MAIL GIVES YOU A WRITTEN RECORD.
- INSTANT E-MAIL LETS YOU COMMUNICATE ONLINE AND CHAT.
- APPOINTMENTS CAN BE MADE BY E-MAIL TO SAVE TIME.
- E-MAIL AND THE INTERNET AVOID EMOTIONAL CONFRONTATIONS.
- REQUEST SPECIAL RATES ONLINE FOR SENIORS.
- REQUEST VARIOUS RATE OPTIONS.
- BE CAREFUL OF CREDIT CARD USE ONLINE.
- E-MAIL MESSAGES CAN BE TRACED.
- TAKE COMPUTER LESSONS.
- ENJOY FREE TRAINING AT LIBRARIES.

CHAPTER EIGHT

SUPPORT GROUPS

Hearing loss can make you feel depressed. Realizing that it is more work for you to hear, you may discover that you tire easily. It is essential that you educate others so that they will understand what is happening.

Friends and family can definitely help once they understand. There are also some wonderful support organizations. In this chapter, I have provided a list of some resources that already exist. It does pay to make connections and look into the organizations that focus on hearing problems. Most support groups are listed online, and many have websites. You can review the website information and discover if you might want to join the organization. Usually membership is inexpensive, and includes conferences, a newsletter, and discounts on products. Some of the organizations have a local chapter. By attending a meeting, you can find others who live in your area. Why reinvent the wheel? Most of the members are happy to share ideas.

Meetings generally have a speaker, and often new information is part of the program. The general organizations and resources listed in this chapter are just some of the options you have. By going online and typing hearing loss or hearing problems, you can do a search for many more resources as well.

The list that follows simply names the agencies, and it is up to the reader to decide which sources to pursue. In short, this is not an endorsement of any organization. It is just a list culled from different sources. In the book called *LIVING WITH HEARING LOSS*, the authors share a very extensive list which is located in Appendix 1 on page 289. I have selected only a few of the resources that they list. By referring to the full text, you can learn about seventy different resources. To find the book use the ISBN NUMBER 0-8160-4140-7. The authors are Turkington and Sussman.

ORGANIZATIONS AND RESOURCES

NAMES and ADDRESSES

1. American Deafness and Rehabilitation Association
P.O. Box 6056
San Mateo, CA 94403
501-663-774 www.adara.org

2. American Society for Deaf Children
1820 Tribute Road, Suite A
Sacramento, CA 95815
800-942-ASDC   www.deafchildren.org

3. American Speech-Language-Hearing Association
10801 Rockville Pike
Rockville, MD 20852
301-897-5700   www.asha.org

4. American Tinnitus Association
1618 SW 1st Avenue
Portland, OR 97201
503-248-9985   www.ata.org

5. Better Hearing Institute
5021 Backlick Road #B
Annandale, VA 22003
800-EAR-WELL   www.betterhearing.org

6. Hear Now
9745 E. Hampden Avenue, Suite 300
Denver, CO 80231
800-648-HEAR   www.leisurelan.com/hearnow

7. Self-Help for Hard-of-Hearing People
76910 Woodmont Avenue, Suite 2000
Bethesda, MD 20814
301-657-2249   www.shhh.org

8. Vestibular Disorders Association
PO Box 4467
Portland, OR 97208
503-229-7705   www.vestibular.org

This list is a sample of some of the support groups that exist. Resources offer human services, programs for all ages, guidance on health and hearing, educational opportunities, conferences, and new legislation. It makes sense to search their websites to see what already exists. Services do vary, but in general they all have valuable information. Usually, they are willing to reply to your questions.

SOLUTIONS FROM CHAPTER EIGHT

- HEARING ORGANIZATIONS SUPPLY FREE INFORMATION.

- ORGANIZATIONS OFFER CONFERENCES.

- GROUPS CAN INITIATE NEW LEGISLATION.

- GROUPS CAN HELP TO ENFORCE FEDERAL LAWS AND POLICY.

- GROUPS CAN INFLUENCE THE MEDIA.

- GROUPS CAN OFFER SOCIAL OUTLETS.

- ORGANIZATIONS CAN MAKE YOU AWARE OF RESOURCES THAT ALREADY EXIST.

- NETWORKING MAKES SENSE.

- SOME ORGANIZATIONS OFFER DISCOUNTS ON PRODUCTS.

- MAGAZINES AND NEWSLETTERS KEEP YOU UPDATED.

- GROUPS MEET LOCALLY AS WELL AS NATIONALLY.

- GROUPS ARE ADDITIONAL SUPPORT TO FAMILY AND FRIENDS.

- GROUPS CAN EDUCATE YOU ON THE LATEST TECHNOLOGY.

- GROUPS CAN BE FUN.

CHAPTER NINE

THE COCHLEAR IMPLANT

The cochlear implant is the newest device for hearing. It is used for individuals who have severe to profound hearing loss. Often when hearing aids no longer are effective, the implant is an alternative. This device converts sounds directly to the auditory nerve. In this way it bypasses the damaged part of the inner ear called the cochlea.

The implant is surgically implanted, and a candidate needs to receive a professional evaluation to discover eligibility. The evaluation is done at a cochlear implant clinic. A group of professionals work together to decide if the patient is eligible. Usually the team includes an ENT surgeon, an audiologist, a social worker, and a psychologist.

The audiologist will test the level of hearing loss. The surgeon will examine the ears and scan the cochlea to be sure that it is suitable for an implant. Also, the surgeon will check to see that there are no ear infections. In the case of children, often others are on the team doing the evaluation. An educational assessment might be added.

In addition, the general health of the candidate is analyzed. The person must be able to undergo surgery. Naturally, in any surgery there is a risk. The implant team will review the results. The candidate must be strong enough to undergo surgery with anesthesia. The surgery usually takes two to three hours, and most hospitals require a brief hospital stay.

The program involves not just the initial surgery, but a rehabilitation period as well. First, the surgery takes place. Then there is a healing period. Once the surgery has healed, then the next step can follow. Cochlear implants have external and internal parts. The internal part is placed under the skin behind the ear. This is implanted during the surgery. Once the surgery is done there is no hearing in that ear. The surgery cuts off any prior hearing that existed. There is a healing period before the next stage. The healing period could be a month to six weeks or more.

The second stage involves connecting the external parts which include a microphone, a speech processor, and a transmitter. The microphone looks like a behind-the-ear hearing aid. It picks up sounds and sends them to the speech processor.

The speech processor is a computer that analyzes the sound signals, and sends them to a transmitter worn on the head behind the ear. The speech processor takes the signals and codes the sounds electrically. The signals are sent to electrodes, and they are transmitted across the skin via radio waves to the implanted device. The electrical signals stimulate the auditory nerve, and then the brain is able to interpret the sounds. It is the brain that must do the interpretation. The normal ears are the microphones for hearing. In the case of the damaged ear, the implant attempts to bypass the nerve endings that no longer work. Cochlear implants have improved the communication skills of clients who have lost the ability to hear.

Naturally, there are risks involved. Surgery could lead to infection and there is no guarantee how effective the implant will be. Also, once the surgery is performed, any partial hearing in that ear is destroyed. The patient needs to know this in advance. The process is time consuming, costly, and there is no way of knowing in advance the total results. On the positive side, many successful implants have been done, and the benefits to children allow them to lead a more normal educational and social life.

Most insurance companies will help pay for all or part of the surgery. So far, the rehabilitation period when the mapping is done is not covered by insurance. This phase is both costly and time consuming. During this period the audiologist tries to work with the patient to see what external connections work best for hearing. In essence, they need to map out a plan for the most effective connections.

This mapping period is costly, and it involves a series of appointments to discover the best results.

The total cost of the implant varies based on where the surgery is done. It is much more expensive than a hearing aid. The cost, which includes the rehabilitation, could be as much as $75,000. Insurance may cover most of the surgery. You need to do some research to find out in advance exactly what is covered by your insurance. Insurance plans vary, and they can differ on what costs they do cover. Get authorization in writing before surgery.

Implant research is ongoing. Presently there are three FDA approved companies in the United States that produce the product, and one or two in Europe as well. Generally, the longer a person has been deaf, the slower the progress. Children as young as 12 months can receive the implant. These children usually do well, and are able to enter special educational programs that foster their hearing development. Some can be mainstreamed into a regular classroom.

Implant surgery does require both research and commitment. There are still problems that need to be addressed. For example, Advanced Bionics, a United States company that produces the equipment, just announced that they have a reimbursement program for vaccination for bacterial meningitis. This program just recently came into effect, and they are hoping to remove any potential problems that could result. New research is ongoing, and each manufacturer will provide information and videotapes in advance to patients. It makes sense to contact the

56

companies to learn your options.

Research has shown that the cochlear implant can help many people. Today there are support groups of implant users and their families. These groups are growing. By sharing information they network and help each other. If you are considering getting an implant, it is possible to go to some of the meetings before you make your final decision. Doing research and getting information before you finalize your decision makes good sense. Don't hesitate to consult with different professionals for a second or third opinion.

So far it does appear that children who have the implant are more apt to be mainstreamed in schools, and they have a more normal social adjustment as well. This new device could be called the bionic ear, since it has had a major impact on hearing problems for humans. Time and research are needed to discover what will work best for the patient. Each case is different, and one must carefully evaluate the risks and rewards to make an intelligent decision.

SOLUTIONS FROM CHAPTER NINE

- RESEARCH YOUR OPTIONS BEFORE AN IMPLANT.

- LEARN THE RISKS IN IMPLANT SURGERY.

- NOTE IMPLANTS REQUIRE SURGERY IN THE IMPLANTED EAR.

- HEARING CANNOT BE REPAIRED ONCE THE SURGERY IS PERFORMED.

- THE SURGERY CUTS ALL NORMAL HEARING IN THAT EAR.

- CAREFUL EVALUATION IS ESSENTIAL.

- A TEAM APPROACH IS REQUIRED.

- IMPLANTS ARE COSTLY.

- CHECK INSURANCE POLICIES CAREFULLY BEFORE ANY IMPLANT SURGERY.

- GET INSURANCE AUTHORIZATION BEFORE SURGERY.

- IMPLANTS REQUIRE TIME AND MONEY AND PATIENCE.

- CHILDREN AS WELL AS ADULTS CAN HAVE IMPLANTS.

- VACCINATIONS TO PREVENT BACTERIAL MENINGITIS MAY BE REQUIRED.

- ATTEND COCHLEAR IMPLANT GROUP MEETINGS BEFORE YOUR IMPLANT.

- GET A SECOND OR THIRD OPINION BEFORE A FINAL DECISION.

- CONTACT THE COCHLEAR IMPLANT MANUFACTURERS TO LEARN ABOUT THEIR PRODUCTS.

- MAKE SURE HEARING AIDS WILL NOT WORK FOR YOU BEFORE YOU DECIDE ON SURGERY.

- WEIGH THE RISKS AND THE BENEFITS CAREFULLY BEFORE YOU MAKE YOUR FINAL DECISION.

- CONTACT PEOPLE WHO ALREADY HAVE A COCHLEAR IMPLANT.

- TAKE YOUR TIME AND DO YOUR RESEARCH.

- CONSIDER FUTURE RESEARCH. AS TIME GOES ON NEW PRODUCTS WILL DEVELOP.

- MAKE SURE BEFORE YOUR SURGERY THAT YOU ARE WILLING TO TAKE THE RISKS INVOLVED.

60

CHAPTER TEN

FUTURE SOLUTIONS

Solutions to hearing problems are increasing. We have all types of hearing aids, assistive-listening devices, and amplified telephones. Cochlear implants are better than ever. Now there are three manufacturers, all producing excellent implant products. Candidates will have to choose which brand to select.

In addition, the eligibility requirements for the cochlear implant have been updated. Today, they are performing implants on children as young as 12 months old. Also, adults even 80 years of age are considering the implant. It is amazing to realize that in just 20 years the implant has had an unbelievable impact on both children and adults.

Professionals are very optimistic about the future for both

hearing aids and implants. Digital super-power hearing instruments can service the hearing-impaired even with severe hearing loss. One major advance in technology is the inclusion of directional microphones. Now this new feature can be found in various types of hearing aids. In the past this feature was only available in the behind-the-ear model.

There are also new treatments for handling small tumors that affect hearing. Today, radiation therapy is an alternative for those unable to undergo surgery. Naturally, it is best to get several medical opinions before deciding what choice is best for you.

As the demand for products and services increases, the supply will increase as well. At some point insurance laws will be updated. Eventually, the cost of hearing aids will be wholly or partially covered by private insurance companies and Medicare. Now there are groups lobbying for these changes in Washington, D.C. Just recently a new task force was appointed to represent the disabled. The focus of their work will include lobbying for the hearing-impaired.

Earmolds for hearing aids are changing. In the future, they will be made from a laser picture of the ear. This information will be e-mailed to the laboratory where they produce the product. Also, new materials are now being used for patients with allergies. Today they can even boil the materials to remove any plastic allergens.

Telephones also offer new models. Visual phones now exist where you can see the person you are calling. Presently, these phones are costly, but with time the price will be lower. Besides the phone, there will be newer communication tools. Right now the e-mail serves a very special function for the hearing-impaired. The service will continue to be updated and improved.

Groups like SHHH continue to lobby for national action in Washington. Bills to amend Medicare coverage are already being explored. Likewise, a strong program is needed to support screening newborn babies for hearing defects. These issues are important, and as time goes on answers and changes will be forthcoming.

The future is open to new technology. We are living in the age of innovation. There are all kinds of possibilities. The purpose of this book is to provide information to the consumer. Try to be optimistic, have a sense of humor, and learn to enjoy life. It is my hope that by reading this book you will discover useful solutions that will open new doors. I have tried to supply many helpful strategies for hearing loss. Be creative and open the new doors to make your life even more enjoyable. It has worked for me, and it will work for you.

SOLUTIONS FROM CHAPTER TEN

- CLOSED-CAPTIONED TELEPHONES.

- VIDEO TELEPHONES.

- LASER-DESIGNED EARMOLDS.

- SIMPLER COCHLEAR IMPLANT PRODUCTS.

- HAIR CELL REGENERATION.

- DIGITAL HEARING AIDS THAT ARE SELF-PROGRAMMED.

- INCREASED INSURANCE COVERAGE.

- INTERNATIONAL INFORMATIONAL NETWORKS ON HEARING DEVICES.

- NEW PRODUCTS THAT YOU CAN READ.

- INTERACTIVE MEDICINE.

- ONLINE EVALUATIONS FOR NEW TECHNOLOGY.

- LOWER PRICES FOR PRODUCTS.

- LOWER COSTS FOR SERVICES.

- ADDITIONAL EARLY INTERVENTION TESTING.

- PROGRAMMED COMPUTER- DISTANCE LEARNING.

- NEW EDUCATIONAL RESEARCH.

APPENDIXES

66

APPENDIX A

HEARING AIDS AND COCHLEAR IMPLANTS

HEARING AIDS

Listed below are some comparisons of hearing aids and cochlear implants. This list will help you with questions that you may have for your hearing professionals. Naturally, each individual will have differences in terms of ultimate device effectiveness. It is helpful to know some of the questions to ask before meeting with your doctors and audiologists.

HEARING AIDS

• You can try different models for comfort and clarity.
• As new technology becomes available you can have new equipment.

- Cost of hearing aids is much less than a cochlear implant.
- No surgery is involved.
- You can adjust the controls on some hearing aids yourself without an appointment with the audiologist.
- Audiologists are available in nearly every location to give you help and advice.
- Easy to maintain most hearing aids. The parts can be replaced if necessary.
- You retain residual hearing for future hearing aid technology.
- Hearing aids do not require surgery.
- Easy maintenance and flexibility for repairs.

COCHLEAR IMPLANTS

- May enable you to hear better on a regular phone.
- Bypasses the cochlea which is probably the source of deafness.
- Is the choice for those who cannot do well with hearing aids.
- Does involve surgical risk.
- Removes any residual hearing in the implanted ear.
- Avoids feedback problems.
- Costs much more than hearing aids.
- Is not always covered by insurance.
- Requires extensive rehabilitation time.
- When removed or if the device fails, the user will not hear in the implanted ear.

- Long-term results of implants have not been established.
- The cost of surgery and rehabilitation can increase with time. It is essential that you receive an accurate statement of the total costs in advance. Request a written price quote. Some facilities will charge more than others, prices vary.
- Research the benefits you may receive from any medical insurance policies. If possible, get this in writing before you proceed.

How much benefit people get from a cochlear implant varies. Some get little more than improved awareness, and some are able to comprehend speech without lip reading. The results are not immediate, and the results do vary. It takes time for the brain to learn to understand and process new sounds.

Cochlear implants do not cure or fix deafness. They provide an improved perception of sound. When the speech processor is turned off, there is no sound. People who have implants are cautioned against contact sports because a blow to the head may damage the housing. Wearing a helmet would make good sense.

It is essential that before any decision is made, that a comprehensive evaluation is performed. Once surgery is done, it destroys any residual hearing in that ear.

Finally, some users have discovered that they are able to use the implant and the hearing aid in the other ear at the same time. The bottom line is it is up to you. Research and discover what will work best your needs.

APPENDIX B

AMERICANS WITH DISABILITIES ACT

This law signed in 1990 guarantees rights to handicapped Americans. As a result of the law, a job cannot be denied a deaf person if that person is qualified for the job. Businesses are required to make accommodations for deaf employees. This could include amplified phones, special services, and possibly even interpreters. In addition, all public announcements funded by the federal government must be closed- captioned.

Today there are management conferences that address the required policies and procedures that are required by law. A new wave of employer liability exists, and even libraries, hotels, restaurants, parks, and public services are required to comply. The key words are "reasonable accommodations" must be made for deaf employees.

As the baby boomers age and develop disabilities, the number of lawsuits will continue to grow. The new wave of employer liability will apply. Naturally, the lawyers will focus on this law, and if someone is fired unjustly, they will take it to court. Constant update on the law will force agencies and institutions to comply, since litigation is costly and cumbersome.

People with disabilities are encouraged to request the appropriate services, since many of the hotels and public places have not complied. Unless they are made aware of the law, they will try to avoid it. There is strength in numbers, and as the numbers increase, so will the demand.

Resources to contact in case of a problem could include a number of agencies. In Washington, the National Information Center on Deafness would be a good resource to guide you. By calling 202-651-5051, you could receive information and resources. The address in Washington is 800 Florida Avenue NE, Washington, D.C. 20002. The website is http://www.gallaudet.edu/-nicd.

SHHH is another national resource for the hard-of-hearing. This organization has joined other consumer organizations to send letters to Congress to fully fund hearing screening programs. By contacting the organization you can discover the latest information on how the laws may have changed. They have a website and can be reached at www.shhh.org. (see p. 49). If necessary, contact your lawyer. Legal help may be required.

To summarize the law, all handicapped Americans have rights for employment, transportation, public services and telecommunications. These rights are guaranteed by the federal government.

APPENDIX C

CAPTIONED TELEPHONES

Just recently I became a participant in a captioned telephone trial. This allowed me to try a new captioned telephone. Since I am delighted with this new telephone, I have decided to add a section to my book describing the product.

This exciting new telephone warrants a separate section in this book, since is it is a breakthrough in telephone communications. I feel that the product is new, innovative, and a winning solution for the hearing-impaired.

HOW DOES THE TELEPHONE WORK?

The telephone looks like a traditional phone; however, it has special features that allow you to hear the other party while you are receiving captions that transcribe the spoken words. The captions are generated by voice recognition technology that allows you to hear and read what the other person is saying.

Telephone users place a captioned call in the same way you would dial a traditional phone. Behind the scenes are specially trained operators at a service center. They transcribe the spoken words in conjunction with voice recognition technology. To activate the system as a caller you simply push a button that says "Caption". A red light will go on to indicate that you are connecting to the Captioning Service. You then dial the number that you are calling, and after a few seconds you will read a message that lets you know the Captioning Service is being connected. The Captioning Service includes a relay operator who dials the number, and you can begin speaking as soon as you hear the other person answer. In case you are unable to hear what they are saying, you can read the dialogue on a small screen located above the numbers on the phone. The dialogue is printed out as they are speaking. The operator does not speak to you, but corrects any computer errors as the dialogue is printed. The captions appear almost simultaneously with the words that are spoken.

This same phone can be used as a traditional telephone as well. The caller simply dials a number and does not push the caption button. The caption feature also allows you to review the conversation by scrolling back on the screen. The conversation remains printed until you hang up the receiver. The phone also has a separate button for volume.

76

When you need amplification, you can press the volume button and the tone control button to adjust the sound.

ANWERING A CALL WITH CAPTIONS

Because the captions are provided by a Relay Service, the person calling you must first connect with the service. There is a special phone number for each state. When connected, the operator prompts you to enter the area code, and the phone number of the person you wish to reach. Then the service automatically dials the phone number. Often it is easier to call the person back. Once you press the caption button, the other party will automatically be connected as well. You cannot be connected to the service in the middle of a call. You must use the service at the beginning of all calls.

The FCC approved the existence of this new service as of August1, 2003. The phone is available only in states that offer Relay Service. Trials are ongoing in different states. So far the phone is not available. I am not sure when it will be for sale and what it will cost. The price of the product has not yet been determined. The product is still in the trial stage.

This phone is ideal for people with some degree of hearing loss. Hopefully it will be available for purchase in the near future.

77

BIBLIOGRAPHY

BIBLIOGRAPHY

BOOKS

Burkey, John. M. *Overcoming Hearing Aid Fears.*
New Jersey: Rutgers University,1959.

Carmen, Richard. *A Consumer Handbook on Hearing Loss and Hearing Aids.* Arizona: Auricle Ink, 1998.

Hunning, Debbie. *Living Well with Hearing Loss.*
New York: John Wiley, 1992.

Jeffery, Lorraine. *Hearing Loss and Tinnitus.*
London: Ward Lock Book, 1995.

Meyers, David. *A Quiet World: Living with Hearing Loss.*
New Haven: Yale University Press, 2000.

Paseoe, Muriel. *Hearing Aids, Who Needs Them?*
Missouri: Big Bend Books,1991.

Romoff, Arlene. *Hear Again, Back to Life with a Cochlear Implant.* The League for Hard of Hearing, 1999.

Turkington, Carol and Allen Sussman. *Living with Hearing Loss.* New York: Checkmark Books, 2000.

BIBLIOGRAPHY

ARTICLES

AARP. *"Consumers Guide to Hearing Aids"*. Washington, D.C.,2000.

Boothroyd, Arthur. *"Hearing Aids and Room Acoustics"*. *THE HEARING JOURNAL*. Vol.56, No. 10, pp.10-17.

Clarion. *"Introduction to the Clarion II Bionic Ear System"*. California, 2001.

Field,D.L. and Haggard. *"Knowledge of Hearing Tactics"*. *BRITISH JOURNAL OF AUDIOLOGY*. 1989, pp.349-354.

Greenlee, Melissa. *"A Second Chance to Hear"*. *GOOD HOUSEKEEPING*. June, 2002, p.72.

Hartling Communications. *"Assistive Products for Deaf and Hard of Hearing People"*. CATALOGUE.

Walski, Chris. *"It's a Hearing Dog's Life"*. *HEARING PRODUCTS REPORT*. March/April,2003, p.26.

Wynne, Michael. *"Sudden Sensorineural Hearing Loss"*. *THE HEARING JOURNAL*. Vol.56, No.7, July, 2003, pp.10-15.

END NOTE TO THE READER

Many thanks for reading this book. Please tell your family and friends to get a copy as well. It will definitely help them. It has been my joy to write this book. If you have additional comments, information, and strategies feel free to share them with me by sending an e-mail to Nshu4@aol.com.

INDEX

Audiologists
   children's needs, 13-16
   cochlear implants, 53-59
Aging
   hearing loss, 1-2
Alarm clocks
   extra loud, 29
Alerting systems, 29-32
Americans with Disabilites Act
   Appendix B, 71
Assistive Listening Devices, 25-34

Basic hearing evaluation, 2-4
Buying hearing aids, 17-23

Captioned telephones
   Appendix C, 75
Children with hearing loss, 13-16
Closed captioning, 28
   Appendix C, 75
Cochlear implants, 53-59
   Appendix A, 67
Cost of hearing aids, 17-22

Digital hearing aids, 19
Diseases and hearing loss, 14
Dizziness, 3

Earmolds, 18-20
Elderly, 1-2
Emotional reactions, 5-11
Evalution, 3

INDEX

Exercise, 6-7

Financial medical expense, 21
FM listening system, 28-29

German measles, 14

Hair cells, 2
Hearing aids, 17-23
Hearing loss, 1-4

Infrared listening systems, 28
Interpreters, 32

Lip reading, 38-39

Ordering forms, 85-87

Pain, 3
Physician, 2-4
Prebycusis, 1-2

Relay services, 26
Research, 61-64
Resources, 30-32, 48-51

Sensorineural hearing loss, 2
Strategies, 35-42

Telephones, 25-27
    Appendix C, 75
Television, 28

Veterans Administration, 21

ORDERING FORM

To order, write to: SLR PUBLISHING, INC.
8310 Excalibur Circle, Unit Q7
Naples, Florida 34108

Make checks payable to: SLR PUBLISHING, INC.

You may also send an E-mail to:
Nshu4@aol.com

All orders must include:

Your name _____

Your address _____

City _____ State _____ Zip _____

Phone _____ E-mail _____

Number of copies _____

Price: U.S. price in U.S. currency: $15 per book plus
$3 for shipping and handling

To order more than one copy, request a price quote.
The buyer pays shipping costs.

For Gift Orders, include:
Name, Address, City, State, Zip Code, Phone, and
Number of Copies.

ORDERING FORM

To order, write to: SLR PUBLISHING, INC.
8310 Excalibur Circle, Unit Q7
Naples, Florida 34108

Make checks payable to: SLR PUBLISHING, INC.

You may also send an E-mail to:
Nshu4@aol.com

All orders must include:

Your name _____

Your address _____

City _____ State _____ Zip _____

Phone _____ E-mail _____

Number of copies _____

Price: U.S. price in U.S. currency: $15 per book plus
$3 for shipping and handling

To order more than one copy, request a price quote.
The buyer pays shipping costs.

For Gift Orders, include:
Name, Address, City, State, Zip Code, Phone, and
Number of Copies.